I0429845

The
Wheat Belly
Solution

The Wheat-Free Guide for Losing Belly
Fat and Boosting Energy

J.C. Collins

Copyright © 2014 J.C. Collins
All Rights Reserved. No part of this publication may be reproduced in any form or by any means, including scanning, photocopying, or otherwise without prior written permission of the publisher or copyright owner.

Limits of Liability, Disclaimer of Warranties & Terms of Use
This book is a general educational health-related information product. As an express condition to reading this book, you understand and agree to following terms. The information and advice contained in this book are not intended as a substitute for consulting with a healthcare professional.

The publisher and authors are not responsible for any adverse effects or consequences resulting from the use of any of the suggestions, or procedures discussed in this book. While all attempts have been made to verify information provided in this book, the author and publisher assume no responsibility for errors, omissions, or contrary interpretation of the subject matter herein. All matters pertaining to your physical health should be supervised by a health care professional

ISBN-10: 1500511471
ISBN-13: 978- 1500511470

DEDICATION

This book is dedicated to those in search of an effective way to lose weight and eliminate belly fat through The Wheat-Free Diet.

CONTENTS

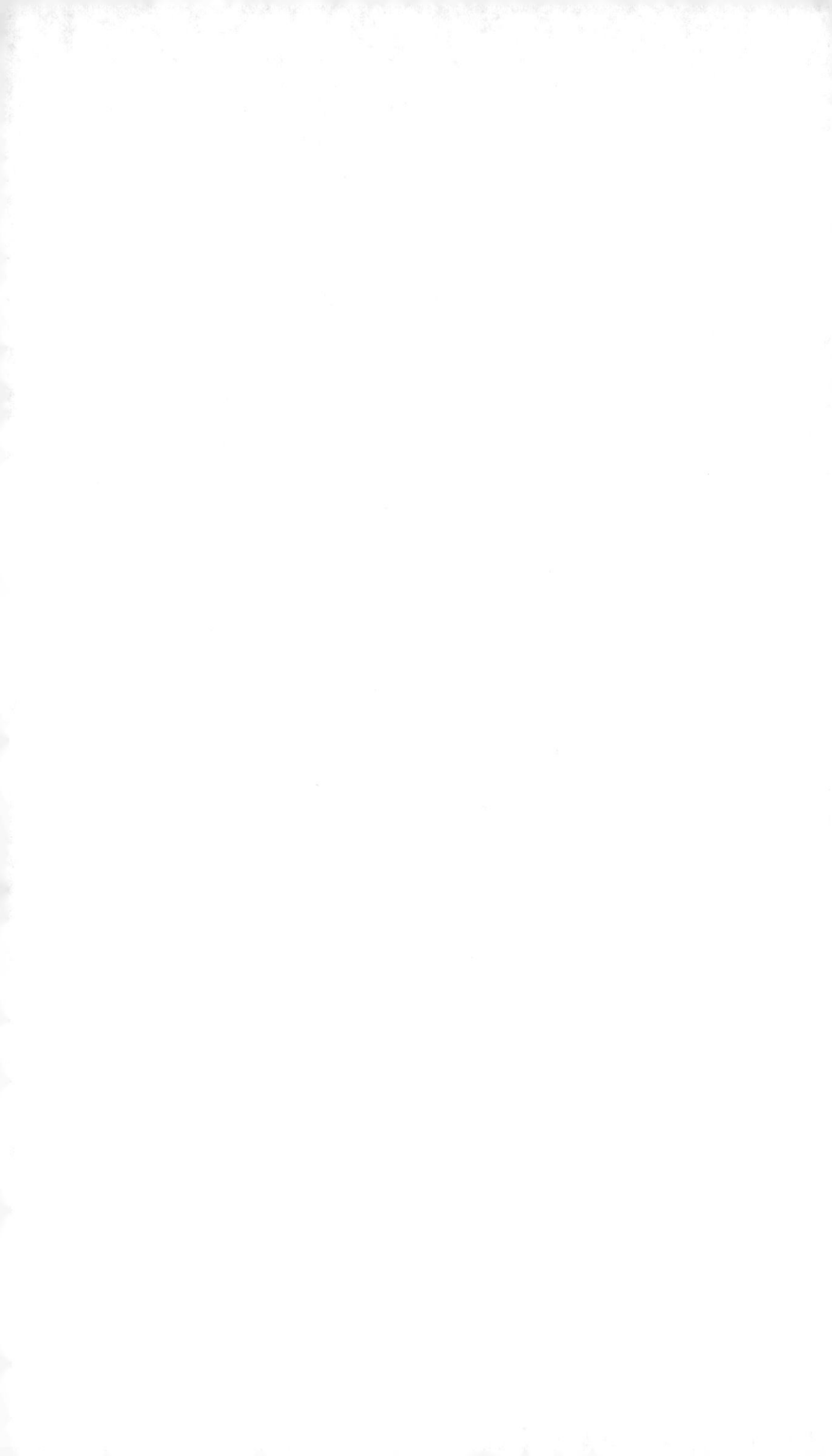

INTRODUCTION

This book contains proven steps and strategies on how to effectively lose weight and eliminate belly fat through The Wheat-Free Diet.

Recent studies have shown that the more fat a person carries around their midsection, the more likely he or she is to develop such life-threatening conditions as heart disease and strokes. This is another reason why many experts believe that all wheat and products with wheat and whole grains in them should be removed from a person's diet.

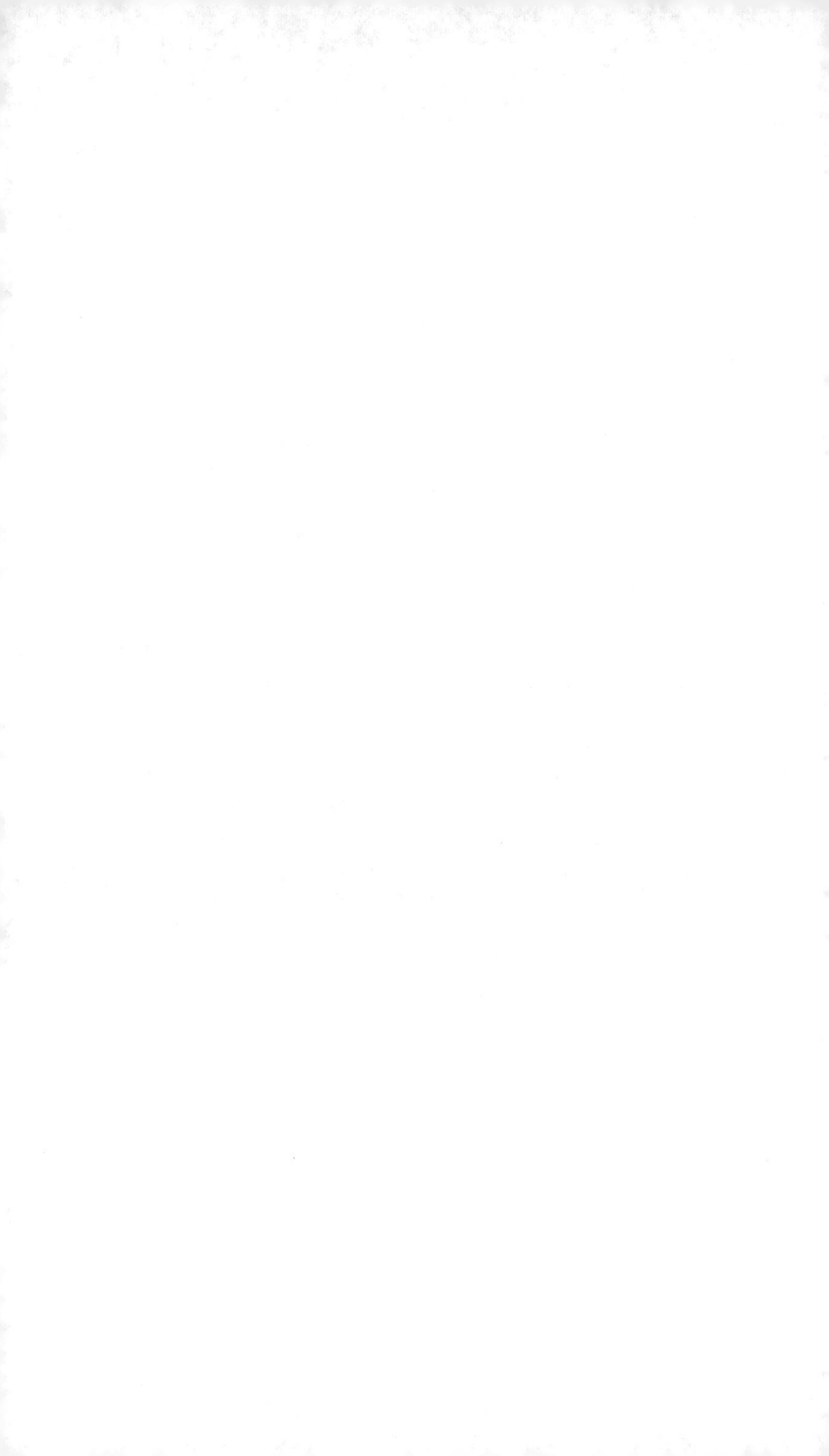

CHAPTER 1 – WHAT IS THE WHEAT BELLY DIET?

The wheat belly diet was first formulated by William Davis, a cardiologist who started a wheat-free experiment after noticing that he was carrying a lot of extra weight around his abdomen. He asked his patients to consume low glycemic food in place of foods made from wheat. Most of his patients lost a significant amount of weight after three months and their blood sugar level also improved. The patients also reported other benefits like increased energy levels, better bowel movement and better breathing.

Dr. Davis' central theory is this: the agricultural business has changed wheat so much in the last 20 years that wheat is no longer the "good grain" that it once was. Today, wheat is a storehouse of sugar and other ingredients that give Americans everything from what Dr. Davis terms "wheat belly." It's also not the result of an American eating binge where we stuff our faces from morning to night with sugar-bearing, fattening foods. The way today's wheat plant is developed and the chemicals used not only to increase a field's yield have resulted in everything from minor rashes to high blood sugar to the "wheat bellies."

Benefits of Eliminating Wheat from your Diet

The Wheat Free Diet is essential for people with celiac disease and gluten sensitivity since wheat can aggravate their condition. People can also experience benefits such as:

- *Improved digestion*

Wheat contains a protein called gluten that is difficult to digest. Gluten becomes sticky when it is wet and it sticks to the stomach lining. This can make it difficult for the body to digest the food and absorb its nutrients. Since gluten stays in the gut for a long time, it can also encourage bacterial growth which can result to constipation, gas and bloating.

- *Generally healthier diet*

Once you eliminate wheat from your diet, you are also eliminating unhealthy processed foods like cereals, bread and sugar-laded cookies. This type of diet enables you to look for healthier alternatives like fruits and vegetables.

- *Prevents bone loss and joint pain*

Some people who are allergic to wheat may not experience any digestive symptom but experience bone loss and joint pain instead. Common symptoms include arthritis and osteoporosis. Studies also show that adults may experience less digestive symptoms than children. Consult your doctor if you experience unexplained joint pain.

- *Weight loss*

Even people who are not after weight loss may experience a drop of unwanted pounds by eliminating wheat from their diet. People who stick with the diet also kept the weight off. People on a wheat belly diet are highly encouraged to consume more lean protein and vegetables instead.

- *Neurological*

Some studies suggest that eliminating wheat can help people achieve better focus and reduce brain fog. It can also improve your mood. Some parents of children with ADHD also say that eliminating wheat from their children's diet can reduce the symptoms drastically. It can even reduce the risk of depression.

- *Reduce inflammation*

Wheat can trigger the release of inflammatory molecules called cytokines which can inflame your body's tissues. This can cause muscle cramping, numb legs and chronic inflammation. Skin inflammation and rashes can also be a sign of wheat intolerance. People with eczema may experience improvement after eliminating wheat from their diet.

- *Improved energy levels*

Gluten may be preventing your digestive system from absorbing all the nutrients and vitamins from the food you are consuming. This can lead to malnutrition and reduce your energy significantly. Many people report feeling sluggish and weak after indulging in wheat products.

J.C. Collins

CHAPTER 2 – HOW TO START THE WHEAT BELLY DIET

Reducing your wheat intake can help your digestion and even decrease inflammation. A wheat belly diet is even more essential for people with celiac disease and gluten sensitivity.

Here are the tips in reducing your wheat intake.

Make a journal

Doctors usually recommend their patients to keep track of their food intake at the beginning of any diet change. This can help you determine if you have gluten sensitivity and other food allergies. Consider maintaining a food journal and recording any reaction that you may have to gluten.

Reduce your wheat consumption

Start reducing your wheat consumption. This can be challenging if you are used to using bread for your sandwiches but you can find alternatives like wrapping your sandwich in lettuce instead of bread.

- During the first few weeks, it is better to reduce the total amount of bread that you consume instead of simply replacing them with gluten free alternatives. Many gluten-free products contain other fillers and may not be able to provide your body with its needed nutrients.

Make it a habit to read labels

- Beware of products that have a long list of ingredients since they are more likely to contain wheat. One of the reasons why consuming whole foods are recommended is that they do not contain artificial ingredients.

Increase your whole food consumption

- Focus on consuming whole and unprocessed foods like fruits and vegetables. You should also increase your protein intake to help you feel fuller without relying on wheat products.

- Also, ensure that you are eating a balanced diet from fruits and vegetables to acquire the nutrients needed by the body. Focus on foods rich in thiamine, folate, iron, riboflavin, calcium and niacin.

Replace your drinks

You should not only be wary of your food intake but your beverages as well. Beer and other soda are made from malted wheat or barley which contains gluten. Try increasing your water consumption instead. If you find plain water too boring then try fruit infused water for more flavor.

J.C. Collins

CHAPTER 3 – LIST OF FOODS TO EAT, LIMIT AND TO AVOID

Here are the guidelines in what food to consume on the diet. These are the foods that you can consume in unlimited quantities whenever you feel hungry.

Foods to Eat

Vegetables

- Most vegetables are wheat free so they are a safe choice for most people. Try to choose organic and fresh vegetables as much as possible. Make sure to wash them with warm water to remove any pesticide residue.

- Eat a variety of vegetables in different colors. Also, vegetables should not only be served during dinner. You can eat them any time of the day. The only vegetable that you should be cautious about is corn and potatoes because they contain starch.

Dairy

- Full fat cheese like cheddar, edam, feta, goat cheese and mozzarella are allowed in the diet.

Fish and shellfish

- Fish like catfish, salmon, tuna, white fish, trout, red snapper, perch, halibut and walleye can be included in your diet. You can also consume shellfish and other seafood including octopus, shrimp, crab, clams and mussels.

Meat and poultry

- Meat is naturally free of wheat as long as you do not include other ingredients like breading. Choose organic meat from grass fed animals. Most organic farms raise their livestock under humane conditions where the animals are given free access to outdoors and are given their natural food.

- Meats that are allowed in the diet include beef, veal, lamb, elk and any wild game. You can also consume chicken, turkey, quail, ostrich and duck.

- You can consume uncured sausages like Canadian bacon, Italian sausage and turkey bacon. However, it can be challenging to find these sausages in a regular supermarket. You may find some in local farmer's market and organic shops. Avoid frying your meat and do not coat them in breading. For the total quantity, only consume the amount that your body needs.

- Make sure to read the label when buying cold meat cuts, sausages and prepared burgers since some meat products are added with wheat fillers.

Fats

- You can use healthy oil generously. Some of the best choices include extra virgin olive oil, flaxseed oil, walnut oil, avocado oil and coconut oil. Organic butter can also be included in your diet as well as cocoa butter.

Eggs

- Eggs are an excellent source of protein. They are also one of the cheapest food options for people on a wheat belly diet. Eggs generally do not contain wheat and can be prepared in many different ways. However, avoid egg soufflés and quiche since they are cooked with crust which may contain wheat.

Nuts and seeds

- Most nuts and seeds can be consumed in the wheat belly diet. You can liberally eat brazil nuts, coconut, hazelnuts, almonds, peanuts, walnuts, pecans and macadamias. Sunflower seeds, pumpkin seeds, flaxseeds and sesame seeds are the healthiest option for seeds. Butters made from these nuts and seeds can also be part of your diet.

Flour alternatives

- You should use wheat and gluten free flour in your baking. Also, you have to beware of 'gluten-free' products that use alternative ingredients like rice starch, potato starch, cornstarch and tapioca starch.

- Wheat belly diet greatly recommends almond flour, chickpea flour, coconut flour, ground flaxseed flour, peanut flour, pumpkin seed flour, and walnut meal. Be sure to drink more water if you consume flaxseed flour since it can expand in your stomach. Also, make sure to store your flour in the refrigerator or freezer to slow its oxidation process.

Herbs and spices

- Herbs and spices can improve the taste of your dishes. You can use herbs like bay leaves, marjoram, parsley, rosemary, sage, tarragon, thyme and parsley. Spices like celery seed, chili powder, cinnamon, smoked paprika, onion powder, ginger, nutmeg, salt, star anise, wasabi and mustard is also safe to use.

- You can also use non sugary condiments like chili and hot pepper. Mayonnaise that is not made from soybean is also allowed. Gluten free soy sauce, salsa and Worcestershire sauce is also allowed.

Sweetener

- You do not have to give up all of sweets if you are on a wheat belly diet. You can use alternative sweeteners like stevia, Splends, xylitrol and erythritol in your food.

Avoid cross-contamination

When you are preparing food, make sure that your ingredients do not come into contact with food that contains wheat. For example, if you use a knife to spread butter into a wheat bread then return it to the butter, the butter will be contaminated. This is more common if you are the only person in your house that follows a wheat belly diet. In these cases, try to have two separate containers, one for general use and one that is wheat free.

Foods to Take in Moderation

You can consume other food in moderation. Aim to consume no more than half a cup of these foods each day.

Dairy

- Other than cheese, you should only consume milk, sour cream, half and half in moderation. Greek yogurt, unsweetened yogurt and other cultured milk products can also be included in your diet. Try to choose dairy products that are in their less processed forms like full fat, unsweetened and without any additional flavorings.

Fruits

- Make sure to wash all fruits to reduce their pesticide and herbicide content. You can also purchase fruits from organic shops. The best fruits recommended for wheat belly diet are berries. You can consume cherries, raspberries, strawberries and blueberries.

- Other fruits like apricots, apples and oranges should be limited for a few slices. You should also limit the consumption of fruits rich in sugar like papaya, mango, banana and pineapple.

- Make sure that you drink 100% natural fruit juices. You can include unsweetened applesauce and fruit butters in your recipes provided that you use them in moderation.

Non Wheat grains

- Non wheat grains should be limited to one half cup or less. These are generally recommended for people with no carbohydrate intolerance and for children who are more tolerable of carbohydrates than most adults.

- Rice and corn should also be limited. Aside from their carbohydrate content, they are also most likely to contain GMO and artificial ingredients so consume them as little as possible. These foods should be fully eliminated if you are experiencing wheat withdrawal symptoms.

Legumes

- You should only consume half cup of legumes a day. Beans like black beans, pinto beans, Spanish beans and kidney beans can be consumed in limited quantities. Remember that baked beans may contain corn syrup, sugar and wheat flour.

- Chickpeas, lentils, dried beans and minimally processed soy bean products can also be tolerated. Peanuts should not be consumed raw. Try to boil or dry roast peanuts as much as possible. Also, read the label to ensure that it does not include hydrogenated oil, wheat flour and sucrose.

Starchy vegetables

- Whole corn and potatoes contains starch so they are best consumed in moderation. Corns should not be confused with cornstarch and cornmeal which is typically excluded in a wheat belly diet.

Beverages

Limit your alcohol consumption to 2 glasses of wine or cocktail or one can of high carbohydrate beer each day.

Foods to Avoid

These are the types of food that you should totally eliminate in the wheat belly diet.

Gluten

- Gluten is commonly found in foods like rye, spelt, wheat, barley, faro, durum and emmer. Foods that contain gluten are wheat bread, pasta, cookies, pies, cereals, waffles, pita, cakes and cupcakes. This means that you should try to avoid fast food as much as possible since it typically uses breading, unhealthy fat and other wheat based ingredients.

- Gluten is also found in some cereals and beverages. These beverages include flavored coffee, herbal teas made from malt, barley and wheat. Vodkas are also distilled with wheat and grains.

- Read the food label to ensure that your food does not contain artificial coloring, fillers and thickeners. These processed foods are usually laded with starch and wheat. You should also be aware of your condiments. Some seasonings, sauces and salad dressings are mixed with wheat flour to thicken its consistency.

- Popular desserts like candy bars, corn chips, dried fruit, ice cream and pancakes and cakes are discouraged in the diet. These sweet treats do not only contain wheat but also excess sugar which makes it high in calories and carbohydrates. Eating these foods can only be detrimental to your weight loss efforts.

Flours

- Wheat flours like bread, pastry and all-purpose flour contains gluten. Cornstarch, rice or tapioca starch should also be avoided. You should also be wary of foods that claim to be wheat free but contains other starch as ingredients.

Some flours like quinoa flour, millet and chestnut flour can be acceptable for children who are not gluten sensitive.

CHAPTER 4- HOW TO MAINTAIN THE WHEAT BELLY DIET

Wheat belly diet and other gluten free diets are getting so much attention from health community because of their proposed benefits. However, to eliminate wheat from your diet, you have to know where it comes from.

Dos and Don'ts of Wheat Belly Diet

Here are some dos and don'ts which can help you eliminate wheat from your diet:

Do: Find healthy foods

- When people are starting a new diet, they usually create a list of foods that they are restricted to eat. While this list can have practical purpose, you should also consider making a list of healthy food which you can consume. The idea is to have as many food alternatives as possible to crowd out the wheat products which you used to eat.

- The transition to wheat free lifestyle can become stressful but having the right mindset can make it a lot easier. It is better to think about the foods that you can include in your diet to avoid the feeling of deprivation.

Dos: Choose food without the ingredient list

- Wheat products like cookies, rolls, bread, doughnuts and cereals are staples for most people. There are even foods that contain long list of ingredients, some of which you can't even pronounce. Stick to buying foods with few or about five ingredients only.

Dos: Keep track of how you feel

- Pay attention to the food you are eating and how you feel after each meal. Going on a wheat belly diet is a significant decision whether you are doing it to control your symptoms or to reduce your weight. Make it a habit to be aware of your body's response to certain food items. What you may discover can help you continue the wheat elimination process.

Don'ts: Fall for the "gluten-free" galore

- The first few weeks of the wheat belly diet can be challenging for most people. Some people find themselves relying on gluten-free labeled foods. Wheat belly diet discourages the consumption of these products since they usually contain the same amount of calories and may even have added ingredients. Eating a gluten-free cookie can help you eliminate gluten but its carbohydrates and sugar content can derail your weight loss efforts.

Don'ts: Feel guilty for asking for alternatives

- Eating outside can present different challenges. Fortunately, most restaurants and food chains have gluten free alternatives. If you find yourself in a place that does not offer any wheat-free alternative, try to focus on consuming protein and vegetables with small amount of starch.

Don'ts: Avoid giving in

- Think of the wheat belly diet as a lifestyle change. No matter how committed you are, there will times and instances where your willpower will be tested. You may find yourself in a birthday party or in your old favorite restaurant. The best way to offset this is to plan ahead. You can pack your own food or eat a light meal before heading out so that you will not be too hungry when you reach your destination. You will thank yourself at the end of the day for sticking to your diet.

Wheat Belly Diet on a Budget

Although gluten free foods are becoming increasingly available for everyone, they are generally more expensive than regular products. However, you do not have to spend too much money to eat healthier meals.

- *Eat foods that are naturally gluten-free*

You do not have to pick up that "gluten-free" bagel which costs three times the regular pastry. Eating fruits and quinoa can be a healthy and cheap option. To save more money, try to purchase these products when they are in season.

- *Enjoy old fashioned meat*

Unprocessed meat is wheat and gluten free. To cut cost and to avoid unnecessary added ingredients, buy meat that has not been marinated or prepared. Most shops use gluten and casein in their meat marinades and dressing. It might take more time, but preparing your own sauce and dips can be healthier and cheaper.

- *Collect coupons*

Collecting coupons can help you save a lot of money in the long run. Make it a habit to clip coupons from magazines and newspapers. Some stores even offer more discounts for bulk purchases.

- *Shop local*

Shopping locally produced fruits and vegetables tend to be cheaper because of the reduced transportation cost. This can also enable you to meet the farmers and ask them about their farming techniques. Some local farmers are actually growing their produce organically but do not certify their products to keep the cost low.

- *Snacking is good*

There is no point in starving yourself. You can munch on healthy snacks like grapes, apples and celery throughout the day. Most nut butters are acceptable in the diet and can be a good alternative to most biscuit fillings.

- *Pasta*

There are many cheap alternatives to expensive gluten free pasta. You can eat rice noodles from Asian markets in limited quantities. Spaghetti squash can also be bought at a

bargain if they are in season.
Simply add salt and roast the pasta for a quick meal. Pasta also has a long shelf life so you can stock a lot for several months.

- *Make your own broth*

You can skip buying expensive gluten free broths and make your own from combining celery, carrots, onion and garlic in a pot of boiling water. Just simmer for few hours and enjoy. Make sure to keep the salt at minimum.

- *List your ingredients*

Listing the ingredients that you need to buy makes it easier for you to stay within your budget. Knowing what you need to buy can also help you estimate the total cost of your purchase.

- *Some dairy is acceptable*

Be careful in purchasing flavored yogurt and milk since they may contain gluten and wheat products. Natural milk and cheese can be consumed in moderation and can be used to add more flavor in your food.

- *Create your own flour*

People who are fond of baking pastries can create their own wheat free baking mix. You can make your own flour from nuts and natural flavorings. Also, try to bake from scratch as much as possible since it is easier than standard baking because you do not have to wait for it to rise.

J.C. Collins

CHAPTER 5 – FREQUENTLY ASKED QUESTIONS

Is wheat really that bad?

-The wheat belly diet states that modern farming is what makes wheat bad for humans. Almost 40 years of genetic research has enabled farms to increase their wheat production but genetically alter it in the process. This results to wheat that cannot be digested properly by the body.

What if I cut wheat but still do not lose weight. Does it mean that the wheat belly diet is not working for me?

-No. This might signify that other factors are preventing you from losing the weight. These factors may include various medications such as beta blockers for hypertension and some anti-inflammatory medications. You may also suffer from iodine deficiency or may be exposed to industrial chemicals. Also, cutting wheat from your diet but consuming more calories in the process can also affect your weight loss efforts.

Why is the relationship between wheat belly diet and losing weight?

-Wheat belly diet claims to help people lose weight because its effect has been demonstrated again and again over the past years. Weight coming from the visceral fat at the abdomen is commonly referred to as "love handles" or "muffin top" is a near-term of "wheat belly". Davis states that wheat contains protein that acts as an appetite stimulator once it is digested. Most people experience a reduction in appetite after few days of eliminating wheat from their diet.

Generally, people who eliminate wheat consumption lose one pound a day for the first 10 days. The total weight loss from wheat belly diet can range from 25-30 pounds in three months. Since eliminating wheat can reduce your appetite, you can easily reduce you caloric consumption by 400 calories a day and experience less cravings.

Many wheat belly recipes use almond flour. What if I am allergic to almonds?

-Almond flour is one of the best flours for people on the wheat belly diet. You can also use other meals from ground pecans, walnuts and golden flaxseed. Coconut flour, chia seed meal and sunflower seed meal are also recommended.

The combination of different flours usually works better than using a single ingredient. For example, combine 1 cup of golden flaxseed, 2 tablespoon of coconut flour and 1 cup of pecan meal. Make sure to adjust the liquids in your recipe to accommodate the different combinations.

So is it the same ad going gluten free?

-Yes. However, do not consume gluten-free foods. Wheat raises your blood sugar level higher than sugar. The foods that can increase your blood sugar higher than wheat includes tapioca starch, rice flour and potato starch. Most gluten-free products include these ingredients. These ingredients contain high glycemic carbohydrates which can be turned into energy very fast.

Any person who eats gluten-free food should think of it as an occasional indulgence.

What foods are mostly recommended in a wheat belly diet?

-The diet greatly recommends eggs, raw nuts, fish, meat and a lot of fruits and vegetables. The diet does not also limit the amount of fat. However, try to use healthy fat from olives, coconut and walnuts.

While it may sound restrictive, living a non-wheat diet is rich and varied. Many people are just used to consuming foods made from wheat. Switching to a wheat belly diet can help you lose weight without even feeling the hunger typically associated with dieting.

If I go wheat free, is there any harm in eating an occasional cupcake?

-Yes, most especially if you are diagnosed with celiac disease and gluten sensitivity. It can also have a negative effect on your health if you usually experience addictive symptoms when consuming wheat. If you find it difficult to stop once you start to eat wheat, then it is better to avoid wheat altogether.

Also, people who removed wheat from their diet may experience symptoms like abdominal cramps, diarrhea and gas once they consume wheat again. The wheat belly diet greatly recommends maintaining a wheat free lifestyle once you started.

Is it practical to remove wheat from my diet is most food products in the market has it?

-Yes. Switching to the wheat belly diet means consuming more vegetables, fruits and meat. The only reason why most food companies include wheat in their ingredients is because it taste good and it stimulates appetite making you crave more of their product.

Following a wheat free lifestyle mean being able to create familiar recipes like cookies without the wheat and sugar.

CHAPTER 6 – WHEAT BELLY DIET SAMPLE RECIPES

Here are some healthy wheat belly recipes to give you an idea on what recipes work.

Pepperoni Bread

2 cups nut flour combination

    2 tbsp extra-virgin olive oil
    2 oz pepperoni, sliced
    1 tsp dried rosemary
    ½ tsp dried onion
    1 cup mozzarella cheese, divided
    2 eggs
    1 tsp dried oregano
    1 tsp dried basil
    ½ tsp dried garlic
    Makes 8 servings

Preheat the oven. Combine the flour and half cup of the cheese. Gently stir in the olive oil and eggs. Whisk to combine. Pour the dough into the baking pan lined with baking paper. Shape into a triangle that is about 10 x 16 inches. Bake for 20 minutes or until the sides are lightly brown. Gently place the pepperoni at the center of the bread then top with the cheese. Roll the narrow end of the rectangle then bake for another 3 minutes. Allow to cook for 4 minutes before slicing into desired pieces.

Nut and Raisin Bars

2 cups shredded unsweetened coconut

¼ cup melted coconut oil
½ cup almond butter, room temperature
½ cup walnut fragments
1 cup whey protein
¼ tsp salt
2 tsp ground cinnamon
1 tsp vanilla extract
½ cup raw pumpkin seeds
½ cup dried raisins
Sweetener equal to ½ cup sugar
½ cup water
Makes 12 servings

Preheat the oven. Mix the cinnamon and coconut in a bowl. Mix to combine. In a separate bowl, combine the coconut oil and vanilla. Add to the coconut mixture then stir to combine.

Spread the mixture on a baking sheet. Spread it evenly in the pan and bake for 5 minutes. Stir using spoon then continue to bake for another 2 minutes or until it is lightly brown. Remove from the oven and place in a large bowl. Add the almond butter, pumpkin seeds, raisins, whey protein, salt, and sweetener and combine well. Shape it in bars then store in the refrigerator.

Strawberry Pie

For the crust:

1 ½ cup pecans, walnuts and almond meal
½ tsp salt
1 egg
1 tsp ground cinnamon
4 oz melted butter
For the filling:
8 oz sour cream
1 tsp vanilla extract
8 oz cream cheese, room temperature
Sweetener equal to ½ cup sugar
For the topping:
1 ½ cups water
Sweetener equal to 1 cup sugar
1 cup rice
1 pack gelatin
6 oz fresh strawberries, chopped
Makes 8 servings

Make the crust by combining the salt, cinnamon, nut meal, butter and egg in a bowl. Grease your pie plate then transfer the dough into the plate. Spread the mixture using a spoon. You can place it in the refrigerator for few minutes if it is too sticky to work with. Use an electric mixer to whip the sour cream, vanilla, sweetener and cream cheese. Pour it into the crust then freeze for half an hour.

Combine the water and gelatin in a saucepan. Allow to sit for 5 minutes and stir until the gelatin is dissolved. Add the chopped strawberries then remove from the heat. Stir in the ice and cool for 30 minutes. Pour the gelatin mixture into the pie and chill for 2 hours.

Chocolate Coconut Tart

2 ½ cups unsweetened shredded coconut

2 tsp ground cinnamon
¼ cup coconut oil, melted
8 oz 100% chocolate
½ tsp vanilla extract
¼ cup almond meal
Sweetener equal to 1 cup sugar
14 oz coconut milk
3 eggs, separated
Makes 8 servings

Preheat the oven and spread oil in the pie pan. Combine the almond meal, coconut, cinnamon, sweetener and oil in a bowl. Transfer the dough in a pie pan then spread using a spoon. Bake it for 10 minutes or until slightly brown. Allow to cool.

Heat the coconut cream and chocolate in a saucepan. Stir until completely melted. Be sure not to overheat. Set aside. Whip the egg whites until soft peaks form. Add the egg yolks, cinnamon and vanilla. Spoon in the chocolate mixture and blend until well combined. Pour the chocolate mixture into the pie shell then bake for another 15 minutes. Refrigerate before serving.

Wheat Belly Pizza

1 cup shredded mozzarella cheese

¼ cup garbanzo bean or coconut flour
1 tsp onion powder
½ tsp salt
4 tbsp extra virgin olive oil
2 cups almond meal
4 tbsp ground golden flaxseed
½ tsp garlic powder
2 large eggs
½ cup water

Makes 8 slices

Preheat the oven. Place the mozzarella cheese in a food processor and blend until its texture resembles granules. Combine the almond meal, garabanzo bean or coconut flour, onion powder, salt, garlic powder and flaxseed in a bowl. Stir in the cheese, olive oil, eggs and water.

Spread the mixture in a baking sheet with parchment paper. Spread olive oil in your hands and shape dough into the desired size. You can use a spoon or spatula to form the crust edge. Bake the pizza for 20 minutes. Remove from the oven then top with your choice of toppings. Add mozzarella cheese, tomato sauce, chopped peppers and onions. Drizzle with olive oil then bake for another 15 minutes until the cheese is melted.

No Bake Cheesecake

4 oz cream cheese, softened

$\frac{1}{4}$ cup Greek yogurt
Sweetener equal to $\frac{1}{4}$ cup sugar
$\frac{1}{2}$ cup chopped pecans
$\frac{1}{4}$ cup heavy whipping cream
$\frac{1}{2}$ tsp vanilla extract
6 chopped strawberries
Makes 4 servings

Blend the cream cheese in a food processor until it is smooth. Add the cream, vanilla, yogurt and sweetener. Add in the chopped strawberries. Blend until the fruit releases it juice. Taste and adjust the sweetener if necessary. Spread the chopped nuts into your ramekins. Use an ice cream scooper to divide the batter equally into the ramekins. Serve immediately or store in the refrigerator for an hour.

Avocado Stuffed Salsa

1 medium tomato, chopped

½ red onion, chopped
¼ tsp cayenne pepper
4 medium avocado, halved and pitted
1 poblano pepper, chopped
¼ tsp cayenne pepper
1 lime
Makes 8 servings

Combine all the stuffing ingredients in a bowl. Spoon the mixture into each avocado halves. Drizzle with lime juice before serving.

A FINAL WORD

You may be wondering what is left to eat once you've removed wheat from your diet. Well, I suggest you be creative with you wheat free choices, extend your food choices from what you are used to habitually eating. When successfully wheat free, you may find that you are eating for breakfast, what you would have in the past eaten for dinner. You will be eating real food, and experiencing all the good effects of truly good nutrition.

There is still a debate out there on whether a wheat free diet really is the best one to follow if you are not wheat sensitive. Many people swear they feel better on a wheat free diet, but how much of this is placebo effect and how much is due to just taking in less refined carbohydrates and sugar? That would make anyone feel better. Many nutritionists believe that reducing processed wheat in the diet and replacing it with whole grains is far more beneficial.

Please Leave a Review

Finally, if you enjoyed this book, please take the time to share your thoughts and post a review on Amazon. It would be greatly appreciated.

That review and feedback will help me improve the content in my books – and make each and every one more relevant and helpful to you.

Thank you again and good luck!

J.C. Collins

www.ingramcontent.com/pod-product-compliance
Lightning Source LLC
Chambersburg PA
CBHW070234290526
45789CB00004B/1616